Myasthenia Gravis

Everything You Need to Know About Myasthenia Gravis, Treatments, and Diet Plans to Lead a Productive Life

By **Cailin Chase**

Copyright 2015 by Cailin Chase - All rights reserved.

This document is geared towards providing exact and reliable information in regards to the topic and issue covered. The publication is sold with the idea that the publisher is not required to render accounting, officially permitted, or otherwise, qualified services. If advice is necessary, legal or professional, a practiced individual in the profession should be ordered. - From a Declaration of Principles which was accepted and approved equally by a Committee of the American Bar Association and a Committee of Publishers and Associations.

In no way is it legal to reproduce, duplicate, or transmit any part of this document by either electronic means or printed format. Recording of this publication is strictly prohibited, and any storage of this material is not allowed unless with written permission from the publisher. All rights reserved.

The information provided herein is stated to be truthful and consistent, in that any liability, in terms of inattention or otherwise, by any usage or abuse of any policies, processes, or directions contained within is the solitary and utter responsibility of the recipient reader. Under no circumstances will any legal responsibility or blame be held by the publisher for any reparation, damages, or monetary loss due to the information within, either directly or indirectly.

Respective authors own all copyrights not held by the publisher.

The information within is offered for informational purposes solely and is universal as so. The presentation of the information is without the contract or any guarantee assurance.

The trademarks that used are without any consent, and the publication of the trademark is without permission or backing by the trademark owner. All trademarks and brands within this book are for clarifying purposes only and are the owned by the owners themselves, not affiliated with this document.

Disclaimers

The information in this book is not intended as medical advice or a substitute for consultation with your healthcare provider. This information should be used in conjunction with the advice of your own healthcare practitioner. Always consult with your physician prior to changing and/or discontinuing medications or diet.

Any trademarks or product names used in this publication are the property of their owners, and are for identification only, and no claim implied by their use.

Myasthenia Gravis

Table of Contents

Introduction	1
What is Myasthenia Gravis?	3
Diagnosis	8
Conventional Treatments	11
Holistic Therapies	16
Homeopathy	21
Diet	24
Cookbook	29
Recipes	31
Conclusion	41

Introduction

Myasthenia gravis is a muscle weakening disease caused by the body's immune system attacking the connection between nerves and muscles. It can be difficult to find adequate information about this kind of autoimmune disease and combined with the tiring and debilitating symptoms this can lead to despair. This book aims to provide you with information on your condition and give advice on how to best look after yourself.

A summary of the kinds of symptoms you can expect when suffering from myasthenia gravis will be displayed, showing its similarities and differences with other diseases that your doctor might suspect that you have contracted. Ultimately, you will gain a greater understanding of the underlying mechanisms behind myasthenia gravis and how this informs diagnosis and management by conventional medical doctors.

Given that autoimmune diseases are generally difficult to treat even when the causes are known, conventional medicine often falls short of its target of treating your condition in full. This book aims to give you a range of holistic alternative therapeutic approaches that have been used by other sufferers of myasthenia gravis. Such methods are known as holistic as they take into account not just the physical disease and you as a physical organism, but also they consider the psychological and sometimes spiritual aspects of suffering from disease. Some of these methods will appeal to you more than others, and you can choose the kind of approach that you feel will best work for you as an individual.

It has been well known for millennia that the health of our bodies is highly influenced the food we consume. Diet plays an incredibly important role in our well-being and the increasingly poor dietary habits of many of us living in the Western world have led to a sharp rise in all sorts of lifestyle-related diseases such as type 2 diabetes. This book aims to evaluate specific dietary factors involved in the development of myasthenia gravis and provide advice to combat them in order to minimise symptoms and get you back to your old self.

What is Myasthenia Gravis?

Myasthenia gravis is an autoimmune condition whereby the immune system for one reason or another attacks the body's own tissues instead of attacking foreign invaders such as bacteria. In the case of myasthenia gravis, this affects a particular component of the connections between nerves and voluntary muscles such as those which control eyelid and limb movement and some of the muscles involved in breathing.

Normally this type of muscle is able to contract when the nerve endings attached to it release a neurotransmitter called acetylcholine. This chemical attaches to specific protein receptors on the muscle tissues found in the area of the connection between nerve and muscle known as the neuromuscular junction. These receptors normally respond to attachment by acetylcholine by setting of a chain reaction which eventually causes the muscle to contract.

In myasthenia gravis, the immune system has developed specific proteins known as autoantibodies which can also attach to the acetylcholine receptors on muscle cells. Their attachment prevents the usual attachment of the neurotransmitter and this prevents the muscle from being able to contract via this mechanism.

The way in which some aspects of the immune system function has great relevance to myasthenia gravis and it is worth having a basic understanding of why this is the case. The autoantibodies which attack the aforementioned receptors are produced by plasma cells which are activated by a type of cell known as a T-helper cell. These cells are in turn activated by antigen-presenting cells which simply put present them with a fragment of a protein shaped like the acetylcholine receptor. The overall result is that the plasma cells develop autoantibodies which directly attack any protein with this shape, including the acetylcholine receptor in the neuromuscular junction.

The thymus gland in your chest, which normally shrinks with age, is responsible for the above process and the maturation of the immune system. As such, removal of the thymus gland has been shown to help some patients with myasthenia gravis.

Acetylcholine is normally recycled within the neuromuscular junction so that it and other compounds can be produced by the cells present. This process is unaffected in myasthenia gravis, which results in all the unused acetylcholine floating around being disposed of. Overall, this means that not only are the muscles less able to respond to normal nerve impulses, they also have less access to the neurotransmitters involved in the first place.

The majority of forms of myasthenia gravis occur due to the attack on acetylcholine receptors, but there are several other types of proteins which can be attacked. The overall mechanism of how this happens is approximately the same and the specific symptoms do not different as a result. As such it is really only necessary to know the names of these proteins. The most important thing to realise is that attacks on said proteins are less common and may complicate definitive diagnosis slightly. These include:

Muscle-specific receptor tyrosine kinase (MuSK)
Lipoprotein-related protein 4

There are several diseases that have similar or related pathological processes behind them, and the presentation of such diseases may mimic that of myasthenia gravis in some cases. This makes diagnosis of one neuromuscular disorder over another rather difficult at times. This can be somewhat frustrating to say the least as the symptoms of such conditions can be rather severe. The tests used to distinguish between myasthenia gravis and other diseases will be discussed in a later chapter.

The symptoms commonly found in myasthenia gravis generally result in an overall fatiguability, whereby physical action cause an increasingly severe muscular weakness. Fortunately, however, this fatigue does resolve itself upon sufficient rest. Typically the following movements elicited b sets of muscle groups are affected:

Eye and eyelid movement
Facial expressions
Chewing
Swallowing
Talking
Neck movements
Limb movements
Breathing muscles (rarely)

These effects are fluctuations in nature but tend to be lifelong. However, treatment is possible and you can go on to lead a perfectly normal life with some adaptations made. Symptoms tend not to progress over time, and on the contrary you may find that symptoms reduce in severity after a period of several years.

Diagnosis is generally difficult as a result of the intermittent nature of the above issues as well as the fact that they may often not be severe enough to be noted upon physical examination by a doctor. Usually the first thing you will notice is that one of your eyelids is drooping, a phenomenon known as ptosis. In some people, they may first notice changes in their speech such as slurring.

As a result of the aforementioned muscle weaknesses, the following symptoms and signs can develop:

Eyelid drooping

Double vision

Unstable walking

Difficulty in movement of arms, legs, fingers and neck

Change in facial expression

Difficulty in swallowing, particular thin liquids

Shortness of breath

Impaired, often nasal, speech

Typically, the symptoms of myasthenia gravis are exacerbated by pregnancy in around one in three women. Fortunately, however, these effects are usually limited to the first trimester and do not have any long term sequelae.

In order to limit the chances of causing a temporary form of myasthenia in the baby, a pregnant mother suffering from myasthenia gravis ought to take immunosuppressant medications. Fewer than 10% of babies have signs of this periodic neonatal myasthenia and most of these respond extremely well to standard treatment methods.

It is all well and good talking about what kinds of symptoms you might expect from myasthenia gravis, but many of us like to know why things happen. Unfortunately, as with many autoimmune conditions, we know how the disease process works but we do not understand as much about why it occurs in the first place. Genetics certainly have a role to play, with familial disposition causing approximately 5% of cases.

There appears to be a link between myasthenia gravis and other autoimmune diseases. It is common for autoimmune diseases to occur together and for different kinds to present in different family members. This would suggest that the underlying mechanism is similar, with the specific bodily tissue being affected being the distinguishing feature of each kind of autoimmune disease. Much of the treatment for these conditions thus overlaps, with dietary changes being a particular aspect where the approach is largely the same no matter what the exact autoimmune disease.

The autoimmune diseases which are most commonly associated with myasthenia gravis are as follows:

Thyroid diseases including Hashimoto's thyroiditis and Graves' disease
Type 1 diabetes
Rheumatoid arthritis
Lupus in its varying forms
Demyelinating central nervous system diseases

Though difficult to live with without adequate support, myasthenia gravis is seldom life threatening in any way. However, in rare cases of myasthenic crisis, the respiratory muscles can be affected which means that you may require assistance with breathing. This usually only occurs upon a trigger in people with already weakened respiratory muscles. Generally this applies to the exacerbation of any symptom or sign of myasthenia gravis and such triggers may include:

Infection
Fever
Adverse reactions to medications e.g. Penicillamine
Stress (physical or emotional)
Extreme heat
Thyroid disease

Getting a Diagnosis

As with many trips to the doctor, a diagnosis is made primarily through physical examination and a series of questions to elucidate the cause of your combination of symptoms. This is frequently backed up with blood tests to confirm the doctor's suspicions. Given that fatigue and muscle weakness can be caused by a huge range of things, not all which have to do with the muscles or nerves directly, it can be difficult for this approach to examination to yield results.

Fortunately, some of the signs of myasthenia gravis such as eyelid drooping and known to many healthcare professionals nowadays with medical schools placing a greater emphasis on such conditions than ever before. It is important to be very specific about your symptoms and any bodily signs you may have noticed so that you can give your doctor as many chances as possible to work out precisely what is going on.

Regardless of anything else, a physical examination will always take place. Owing to the intermittent nature of the symptoms and signs of myasthenia gravis, as well as the fact that they may not be severe enough at the time of investigation to be elicited during a purely physical examination, it is possible to miss the correct diagnosis completely initially.

The physical examination will focus on the level of fatiguability of your muscles, in particular looking at how you perform in the following tasks:

Looking upwards and sidewards
Looking at your feet while lying on your back
Deep knee bends
Walking on the toes and heels
Keeping the arms stretched out

Sit-ups

Your performance in the above examination ought to be enough for your doctor to undertake some blood tests, looking for autoantibodies of the nature described earlier in this book. Firstly the autoantibodies against the acetylcholine receptor are sought, but a positive result does not always occur in myasthenia gravis. It is also possible to get a positive result for the MuSK protein with or without acetylcholine receptor autoantibodies.

A more sensitive test, though not as specific as a positive blood test, involves the use of repetitive nerve stimulation. Individual muscle fibres are detected and then tested using a thin electrode which can detect the decreased activity of the muscle due to its loss of sensitivity to acetylcholine-based nerve impulses.

A simpler test that can be done is the ice test, which as you might expect involves placing an ice pack on a set of muscle groups. In cases of myasthenia gravis, weakened muscle groups are seen to improve in strength. This is thought to be due to the lower temperature adversely affecting the activity of enzymes, acetylcholinesterases, which usually break down neurotransmitters. The result is that more acetylcholine is present in higher than usual concentrations to cause the desensitised muscle to contract more effectively.

When the above tests have failed to get you a definitive diagnosis, your doctor may recommend an edrophonium test. This involves the administration of drugs which block the breakdown of acetylcholine by acetylcholinesterase. This causes the temporary relief of muscle weakness and in particular that of the eye muscles.

It was mentioned earlier in this book that the thymus gland, to do with development of your immune system, can be involved in the onset of myasthenia gravis. As a result, you may often have to undergo a chest X-Ray in order to rule out any issues with the thymus gland. Alternatively, an MRI or CT scan might be used to get a 3D picture of the thymus to confirm the lack of presence of abnormal growth of the thymus. Removal of this gland may be indicated in some cases.

If you experience any trouble with breathing your doctor will conduct a pulmonary function test to monitor how effective your breathing is. Advice can then be given about what to do improve your breathing and any assistance you require will be made clear at this point. Hospitalisation is rare, but occasionally is for the best until your breathing improves.

Most diagnoses of myasthenia gravis are made without the use of most of these tests, and it would be very rare not to have a definitive diagnosis after having gone through all of these tests. It can be daunting to have to go through any of these tests, but it is important to know that the risks associated with them are really minimal and once you have your diagnosis you can start making steps in a positive direction. The remainder of this book will look at how you will be treated by conventional medicine and will examine a range of holistic therapies which may like to try as an adjunct to your treatment.

As diet has been shown to have a strong influence on autoimmune diseases in general, there will also be a section on dietary and lifestyle advice to enable you to make the best choices to improve your health and quality of life.

Conventional Treatment

Medication

The most common and most effective form of treatment given by your doctor will be one or another medication of the same kind often used for diagnosis of your condition in the first place. This group of drugs is known as acetylcholinesterase inhibitors, and they function to prevent the breakdown of the neurotransmitter acetylcholine. The subsequent increase in concentration of this neurotransmitter allows the muscles affected to be more likely to be stimulated, resulting in stronger muscles that are more likely to be able to complete daily tasks and less likely to be too fatigued to do so.

The most common of this group of drugs are neostigmine and pyridostigmine. These are commonly taken around half an hour before eating to facilitate the chewing of more solid foods. They tend to be started at a low dose and increased until an optimal level of symptomatic relief is attained.

As with all pharmaceutical medications, side effects can and do occur. Most commonly, acetylcholinesterase inhibitors have been known to cause sweating and diarrhoea. This is because acetylcholine is present elsewhere in the body and functions in these places as a neurotransmitters also. These symptoms can be combatted with the use of atropine, but this drug has side effects of its own so it is always important to be aware of the effects of combinations of drugs, including herbal and over-the-counter remedies.

Another category of medications, usually used in immune-mediated forms of myasthenia gravis, is immunosuppressant drugs. These come from a variety of chemical origins and as such each act in their own way to suppress the immune system and dampen down the effects of autoimmune disease.

Such drugs include:

Steroids such as prednisone
Ciclosporin
Mycophenolate
Azathioprine

These drugs have a global effect on your body and their effects are varied and multiple in nature. Their mechanisms of function tend to take weeks or sometimes months to have the full intended effect. They are strong drugs which work to fundamentally alter the way your immune system is balanced and will only be used if there is no other alternative from a pharmacological point of view. Generally speaking, most people will be treated with one of these drugs plus one of the acetylcholinesterase inhibitors.

In severe cases where your life may be at risk the autoantibodies are physically removed from your bloodstream by means of plasmapheresis, which employs a form of filtration of your blood outside of the body. In addition, special proteins known as immunoglobulins can be administered into your veins in order to bind to and thus inactivate the autoantibodies.

This kind of drastic measure will only last for a few weeks as the immune system is continually producing new cells and proteins, but it will be enough to get you through the worst of the exacerbations of your condition.

Many investigations into drugs which directly modulate the immune system and its development of antibodies against components of the neuromuscular junction are under way. It may be possible in the future to prevent the immune system from further affecting the muscles in the way in which they do in myasthenia gravis.

Surgery

Rarely, surgery may be indicated in cases of myasthenia gravis. Owing to the immune system component of the disease, the thymus gland is often implicated in development of this and other autoimmune conditions. If any abnormal growth of the thymus gland is detected then its removal is indicated.

This is seldom performed unless there is a risk of such abnormal changes to the thymus spreading around the body. Some patients note an improvement of their symptoms after removal of the thymus, but this is a rather hotly disputed area of medicine at the current time.

Physical Advice

In additional to the usual pharmacological treatments that you might expect modern medicine to offer, a range of physical advice is offered by doctors in order to help you to minimise the impact of the effects of myasthenia gravis on your life.

You will be educated as to the nature of myasthenia gravis, particularly its fluctuating, intermittent nature. Exercise is generally encouraged but only within the limits of your abilities, owing to the fatigue that will result from over exertion. Frequent rest when gently exercising is likely to have the most benefit to you.

More specifically, for those myasthenia gravis sufferers who have breathing involvement, a home breathing exercise program is often promoted. This involves learning how to breathe while relying on your diaphragm which is composed of a different kind of muscle to that affected by your condition. You may also be encouraged to practice breathing it pursed lips.

A particular kind of exercise known as interval-based muscle therapy has been shown to have a beneficial effect on several aspects of breathing, including: endurance, breathing pattern, chest wall movement and muscle strength. The combination of these and other exercises with a change in diet may help you to further reduce the effect of your symptoms and help you to lead as much of a normal life as possible.

It is important to realise your limitations and prepare for possible issues that might arise, particularly around the home. It may be advisable to install bars in places such as staircases and bathrooms in order to facilitate your movement around your living space during exacerbations of your condition.

You may find it useful to employ battery-powered devices instead of their manual equivalents in order reduce the chances of muscle fatigue. This may be most appropriate for culinary activities such as whisking or for hygiene practices such as tooth brushing. You could purchase an electric whisk and toothbrush respectively. There are many electrically powered tools and devices that you can make use of to conserve as much energy as possible at all times. You may find that this has a significant on your overall quality of life.

If you find that you suffer from double vision when your eye muscles are weakened, then you might find it beneficial to wear an eye patch. This will prevent the effects of double vision as only one eye will be exposed to any visual stimuli, resulting in seemingly single vision.

While initially you may feel awkward or embarrassed, it is actually quite common for people to have to wear such patches for periods of time. There are all sorts of support groups available to turn to if you need some reassurance and a confidence boost. These include groups specific to myasthenia gravis or autoimmune diseases, as well as those for people with eyesight problems.

You know your own body the best, and over time you will develop your own ideas of what works best for you in order to maintain the highest quality of life that you can. You will learn to plan activities according to the severity of your symptoms at a given time, and you'll be able to adjust things as appropriate.

Holistic Therapies

Despite the success of modern medicine in treating many diseases, particularly infections, there are some things that pharmacology simply cannot do. Modern medicine is often guilty of treating patients as simple physical organisms, ignoring the psychological and spiritual aspects of humanity. In short, modern medicine does not tend to consider the patient as a whole being.

The belief of holistic approaches is that to treat a disease as a whole, you must be able to treat the person as a whole being. Holistic therapies differ in their approaches but their principles tend to be similar in terms of this kind of belief. You may find that holistic options can treat an aspect of your illness, be it physician or otherwise, than modern medicine simply cannot.

All alternative therapies should be discussed with your doctor before undertaking them to ensure that they will not adversely affect your medication regimen. Conventional doctors are increasingly aware of holistic and alternative approaches to treatment and may even suggest a particular approach to use as an adjunct to their own therapy options. This in particular applies to the advances made by nutritional sciences in the form of the autoimmune protocol diet.

Herbal Medicine

Before modern society developed, we relied on our understanding of the uses of many natural medicinal herbs and plants. We tend to use pharmaceutical medication to treat our ailments, but it is worth remembering that most of these medicines were first derived from plant sources. It is likely that our ancestors would have made use of such plants, and in many cases there is documented evidence of such use. This is true of many of the most commonly used medications such as aspirin, which was originally derived from willow bark and was mentioned by the great Ancient Greek physician Hippocrates.

Given the pharmaceutical qualities of many herbal supplements, it is paramount that you discuss their use with a doctor. This is of particular importance in the case of a condition such as myasthenia gravis as you are certain to be taking prescribed or over-the-counter medications of several kinds.

Despite the awareness of the potential efficacy of many herbal remedies, there is not always enough empirical evidence to suggest that their use is worthwhile. That said, there are definitely some herbal remedies that have traditionally used in the treatment of cases of muscle weakness such as is the case in myasthenia gravis.

Nux vomica is the dried seed from the ripe fruit of a plant that is found in South East Asia. It is traditionally used for muscle weakness but empirical studies are currently lacking. This may be of some help to you, but it is very important to be aware that due to the strychnine content of these seeds adverse reactions are not all that uncommon.

Astralagus is an immune system stimulant often used in combination with other herbs in traditional Chinese medicine. It is increasingly popular in the United States and may be of some use in improving symptoms of myasthenia gravis. Once again though, scientific evidence is lacking as of the present moment so this kind of herbal treatment should be used with caution. If you do decide to take astralagus, you should inform your doctor as there have been reports of decreased effectiveness of immunosuppressants upon taking this herbal supplement as well as adverse effects in patients with diabetes, high blood pressure and kidney issues and in those taking anticoagulants.

The various kinds of reishi mushrooms promoted in the traditional Chinese medical system have also been purported to have a positive effect on muscle weakness associated with myasthenia gravis. However, it is not advised for use by people who suffer from diabetes or high blood pressure. It is also contraindicated if you are taking anticoagulants. In this way it should be treated with the same caution as astralagus.

Herbal practitioners may advise the inclusion of turmeric and ginger in your diet owing to their anti inflammatory and antibacterial properties. It is well recognised that gut inflammation and overall digestive health has a significant impact on the health of your whole body. This is of particular importance in terms of autoimmune disease as there is an increasingly large amount of evidence to suggest that the effects of autoimmune diseases are exacerbated by the inclusion of certain foods in our diet. Fortunately, this also works in the opposite direction, with anti inflammatory foods having a positive effect on the body. Further dietary alterations will be discussed in a separate section due to their great importance.

Traditional Chinese Medicine

Traditional Chinese medicine has been used for thousand of years in its country of origin and its treatment modalities involve aspects of herbal medicine with the use of adjunct such as acupuncture. A short description of the main beliefs behind this kind of therapeutic approach is necessary in order to understand exactly why a particular therapy might be advocated by traditional Chinese medicine. One thing to say for sure is that it is a very holistic approach, taking into account every possible aspect of your being.

Traditional Chinese medicine has truly philosophical basis as it focuses on our way of life and the idea of there being a fundamental duality in nature. Each phenomenon in the

world is represented by two opposing aspects known "yin" and "yang". Generally speaking, rest or calmness correspond to "yin"
whereas activity and rashness correspond to "yang". This concept of balance in all things is understood alongside the concept of a five element system in nature.

The five elements of nature are represented by Wood and Fire as the mostly "yang" elements, Water and Metal as the more "yin" elements and Earth as a balance between the two. Each organ is considered as part of a larger, functional system rather than as a simple collection of tissues working as a whole.

It is considered that each organ system is related to each one of these elements and health is assessed in terms of the effects of yin and yang
on a person's life force or "Qi". This concept is somewhat alien to most of us in the West, but that is not a reason to discard traditional Chinese medicine as an effective way to treat a variety of diseases.

It is believed that disease states are caused by an imbalance in this Qi and the channels, or meridians, in which it collects. There are generally four theories as to the underlying cause of myasthenia gravis in terms of traditional Chinese medicine, and these are as follows:

Reduced Qi in the stomach or spleen
Reduced Yang in the kidneys or spleen
Reduced Yin in the kidneys or liver
Reduced Qi in the blood

A practitioner of traditional Chinese medicine will come to one of these conclusions in the case of myasthenia gravis, and any treatment given will be used with the purpose of bringing balance back to the body.

Acupuncture is frequently used as an adjunct to any herbal remedies with the aim of stimulating the meridians and properly connecting the internal organs to the limbs. The ultimate effect of this is believed to be the activation of Qi and the blood and the regulation of yin and yang to strengthen the tendons, bones and joints.

Acupuncture can be used on the face and ears as well as on the body in general, and this specialised approach is actually more likely to be indicated in myasthenia gravis. In particular, drooping eyelids are treated with acupuncture targeted at the face.

It is not generally considered a painful procedure, but you may experience some strange sensations and perhaps some discomfort when first undergoing acupuncture. Also symptoms are often expected to get slightly worse before they begin to improve.

Though empirical evidence of the precise effects of such therapeutic modalities is lacking, acupuncture in particular has been reported to reduce stress levels which in itself has a hugely positive effect on chronic disease. The influence of the mind over the body in this respect should never be underestimated.

Homeopathy

Homeopathy is based on the idea that any causative substance can also have the opposite effect, that is to say a curative effect. The central tenet of homeopathy as a treatment modality is the idea that like cures like. Homeopathic remedies are formulated by diluting a purported active substance in distilled water until there is almost nothing of the original substance left. This process of succussion is believed by practitioners of
homeopathy to have the effect of magnifying the properties of the original ingredient.

The very concept of homeopathy has been placed under great scrutiny by the medical profession. It is increasingly unlikely that any conventional doctor will recommend it as an effective treatment method by your conventional doctor. However, if you feel that it is something that is worth trying out then there are no documented cases of any harm being caused as a result of such therapy when prepared as described above.

There are several compounds that have been suggested for use in the treatment of muscle weakness in the case of myasthenia gravis. However, as with homeopathy itself, there is no empirical evidence to suggest that it will be effective. That said, lack of evidence is not always the same thing as lack of effect, and as such you may benefit from such treatment in other ways. These compounds include:

Alumina (prepared from aluminium oxide)
Conium (prepared from hemlock)
Gelsemium (prepared from yellow jasmine)

None of these compounds should be consumed in any form except as part of a properly prepared homeopathic remedy. In particular, hemlock is extremely poisonous and is what killed the Ancient Greek philosopher Socrates.

Biofeedback

The ultimate aim of this approach is to gain a greater awareness of the physiological processes going on inside your body in order to consciously affect them. It has been shown that it is possible to manipulate many measurable aspects of physiology including muscle tone. Training is undertaken initially by using a measuring device to detect muscle tone and then learning to alter this.

Eventually this process should be a completely conscious act such that you do not require the measuring device in order to be aware of the changes that you are making to muscle tone. Some studies have shown that it is in fact possible to control individual motor units within muscles. This is believed to have applications in many neuromuscular diseases.

Yoga and related breathing exercises known as pranayama are essentially methods of biofeedback. As such, you don't necessarily have to use this treatment modality with sensor machines or anything else. Yoga has been practised for millennia and it is a gentle form of exercise and is suited to and can be adapted for people with muscular weakness and rapid fatiguability.

Guided Imagery

Guided imagery is a form of therapy that is used in conventional and alternative medicine alike, and it involves the use of mental imagery for the purpose of healing or problem solving. It also involves learning breathing and relaxation techniques in order to control stress levels. This in itself can be very useful when dealing with chronic diseases, aside from any direct effects it may have on your condition.

Guided imagery can also be conducted alongside music for greater effect. Ultimately, the kind you choose highly individual and should be particularly suited to you as a whole person for the best effects to take place. It is often considered as a form of hypnotherapy, and as with conventional hypnotherapy it does not necessarily work on every single person who tries it.

Hypnosis

Hypnosis involves being put into a kind of trance by a skilled practitioners. In the past, it was treated with much scepticism by the modern medical community but it has been increasingly noted that it is effective as part of treatment for a number of different diseases.

While hypnosis is not necessarily therapeutic in and of itself, it can be used as an effective adjunct to other therapies that you may want to use. It is particularly useful when it comes to dealing with the psychological aspects of coping with a long term illness.

Diet

It has long been believed that all disease begins in the gut, and with autoimmune diseases in particular this is increasingly seen to be the case. Inflammation and imbalance of naturally-present gut bacteria has been shown to have a significant effect on the progression of autoimmune diseases such as myasthenia gravis. By making some simple dietary changes you can greatly improve your quality of life.

There are various dietary approaches that have been researched both empirically and anecdotally with the purpose of finding a dietary solution to autoimmune disease. One particular approach known as the autoimmune protocol has been shown to be especially effective in minimising the symptoms of myasthenia gravis as well as other autoimmune diseases. This dietary approach and some specific alterations for specific aspects of myasthenia gravis will be demonstrated through a collection of recipes at the end of this book.

Omega-3 fatty acids are commonly found in oily fish such as tuna and mackerel as well as in nuts and seeds such as walnuts and flaxseed. This type of fat is particularly useful in ensuring that the balance of different fats you consume is overall anti-inflammatory. A reduction in gut inflammation will improve your absorption of nutrients and will prevent the contents of your gut from over stimulating your immune system and thus leading to disease.

Just as there are some fats which are beneficial, there are others which have an overall detrimental effect on your health. One such group of fats is known as trans-fats. These are fats and oils which have been chemically altered from their natural state, and the changes made mean that the compound consumed has a more inflammatory effect on your body. This inflammation has exactly the opposite kind of effect compared to anti-inflammatory effect of omega-3 fatty acids. As such, trans-fats should be avoided in order to limit stimulation of the immune system.

Your nerves and muscle rely on a number of electrolytes in order to function properly. These include potassium, sodium and calcium amongst others. Particularly relevant to myasthenia gravis is the link between low potassium levels and fatigue. Diarrhoea as a result of your medication may also lead to potassium deficiency. Therefore it is very important to ensure that your diet contains lots of fruits and vegetables high in potassium. Such foods include bananas and lean sources of meat such as chicken and turkey. Potassium is found in reasonable quantities in most fruits and vegetables but it is particularly abundant in those mentioned above.

Many of us are intolerant of lactose without even realising it. After all, in the grand scheme of things animal husbandry and thus the consumption of dairy products is quite a recent phenomenon. As modern humans evolved we likely did not consume dairy products at all, and even if we did it would have constituted a tiny proportion of our overall food intake.

Consumption of fresh dairy products may cause an increase in gut inflammation and thus adversely affect your immune system and exacerbate the symptoms of your condition. If you consume dairy products at all, it would be best to stick to fermented milk products such as kefir or yogurt. The live bacterial cultures in these products are actually beneficial for your immune system overall as a result of their balancing effect on the microbial flora of your gut. It may be wise to cut out these products completely at the beginning of adopting a diet focused on treating autoimmune conditions. You can always add food groups back in to your diet one at a time to work out what adversely affects you and what does not.

Meat can be particularly difficult to chew and this problem is made far worse by the jaw muscle fatigue induced by myasthenia gravis. If you consume meat, it would be advisable to stick to leaner, softer meats such as chicken and turkey. Fish is also a great food to add to your diet, particularly those high in omega-3 fatty acids as mentioned earlier in the chapter.

Additionally, protein in any form should be limited. It would be best to limit protein intake to only around 10% of your caloric intake. This can be difficult but good sources include beans and nuts. These might be initially avoided when embarking upon a diet directed to assist the body in fighting autoimmune disease, however they may later be consumed if your body tolerates them.

Many sufferers of myasthenia gravis are often prescribed a steroid such as prednisone by their doctors. While useful for their anti-inflammatory effects steroids have a global effect on the body. Some of these effects can be counteracted by making the necessary alterations to your diet.

Steroids promote loss of bone density, or osteoporosis. This increases your chances over time of fracturing the affected bones. Calcium is a very important mineral for maintaining bone density and should be consumed in high amounts in order reduce the effects of steroid use on bone. If you find yourself unable to tolerate dairy products, then it is important to find viable alternative sources of this vital mineral. Fruits and vegetables high in calcium include broccoli, kale, figs and oranges. Other foods high in calcium include sardines, salmon and almonds.

Steroids also have an effect on vitamin D production which also affects calcium regulation within the body and thus bone density amongst other things. Aside from getting more sun exposure, there are a few good sources of vitamin D in the diet. These include oily fish and eggs.

One of the major things first noticed by people with myasthenia gravis is that they find it hard to chew and swallow for long periods of time. Therefore it is very important to adapt your diet to include predominantly soft foods that require minimal chewing. This is particularly relevant in terms of meat consumption. Many meat products are difficult to chew and you ought to choose softer products such as poultry or fish. Furthermore, foods can be eaten with sauces to lubricate them as they are swallowed.

At the other end of the spectrum, it can also be difficult to swallow thin liquids. This can be helped by adding a thickener to thin liquids. You could use many different foods products to thicken liquids; there's no need to resort to any kind of chemical thickener unless you want to. Such thickeners might include rice cereal, tapioca or gelatin.

Exercise

As promoted by conventional medicine, exercise is a great way to increase your endurance and limit the effect of muscle weakness. There are many different approaches to exercise when it comes to working out while living with conditions such as myasthenia gravis, but it is generally considered a good thing to exercise within your limits in order to promote well-being. It is particularly important in countering the side effects of medication and the consequences of a life consisting of reduced activity on account of a chronic illness.

Strength training within reason is important for several reasons. Firstly, the use of steroids in the treatment of myasthenia gravis causes loss of bone density over time, a condition known as osteoporosis. This can be combatted by dietary means such as increasing calcium intake, but also by strength exercises which are proven to increase bone density.

Due to the decreased average level of activity as a consequence of your condition you may find that it is harder to maintain a steady weight. Exercise can help you to maintain a high metabolism and reduce the risk of weight gain. In addition your stamina will improve in spite of your condition and you'll find yourself able to conduct your daily activities with a lessened need for rest breaks.

A gentler way to exercise that is very useful in muscle weakening conditions such as myasthenia gravis is to focus on stretching as in yoga. While you may not be able to perform some movements usually associated with such exercise, there is plenty that you can still do and a positive attitude in this respect works wonders. You'll be sure to improve your flexibility and range of motion, something which is very useful when finding alternate ways of doing things such as lifting objects.

Obviously there will be certain limitations when exercising if you suffer from myasthenia gravis, but there are steps you can take to get the most out of your exercise and safely reap its rewards. You should always assess your overall weakness with your doctor before embarking on any new kind of exercise to ensure that it is suitable for you. If you focus on exercises on or near the ground then this may be a good way to avoid falling. After all, you can't fall over if you're already on the floor.

Given the inherent risks of exercising when you have particular physical limits, it is important that you do not push yourself too far. It is good to set yourself a challenge, but make sure that it is a manageable task. It is highly advisable to exercise only in the presence of another adult so that if you need help then you can easily get it.

Aside from the physical benefits of exercise, you will most likely notice an increase in your mood which is invaluable when learning how to cope with a chronic illness. This mood increase is partially due to the release of endorphins, your body's natural "feel good" hormones.

Cookbook

The autoimmune protocol, which is advised to be followed by everyone who suffers from autoimmune disorders, follows all the principles discussed in the previous chapter. It is based on a diet that is directed at minimising inflammation and reducing the overstimulation of the immune system. While autoimmune conditions do not necessarily vanish, their symptoms can be reduced significantly if you follow these principles.

Generally speaking, for the recovery of your immune system it is best to avoid grains as they often contain gluten. Legumes, that is to say beans, should also be removed from your diet in the beginning as they contain anti-nutrients which will prevent your gut from absorbing the kinds of nutrients that you need to recover your health. All products containing alcohol and added sugar should be eliminated as they are not really useful to your body and are essentially empty calories, not to mention the fact that they have an overall inflammatory effect on your gut.

Though usually a great source of protein, eggs should really be avoided if you have an autoimmune complaint like myasthenia gravis because some of the protein components of the egg white can pass through the gut lining intact. The cells of the immune system may react to these proteins and cause an exacerbation of your symptoms. You can reintroduce eggs into your diet at a later point in time and see if your body tolerates them well.

In general, nuts and seeds ought to be avoided, as well as their oils, as they are high in the same kinds of anti-nutrients as grains and legumes. You could use coconut or olive oil instead, as well as limited quantities of animal fats. Nuts and seeds also tend to have an inflammatory effect on the body. The only exception that you may wish to make is for walnuts and flaxseed, if you are able to tolerate them, as they have an omega-3 to omega-6 fatty acid ratio which is beneficial for reducing inflammation.

Such a drastic change in diet may seem overly restrictive, but there are many alterations you can make to classic recipes in order to make them suitable. The effects of such a diet on your symptoms may well be significant enough that you'll be happy to continue with this way of eating indefinitely.

It is always possible to slowly reintroduce some of the food groups you have eliminated in order to find out which ones are tolerated well by your body and which ones are not. This can be easily done, but should be done slowly with one food at a time so that you can make a fully informed decision about which foods you would like to permanently reintroduce into your diet.

Generally the least likely foods to cause your symptoms are eggs, seeds, nuts, butter and vegetables. Wait a few days after reintroducing a food and note any symptoms over this time. You can then be sure about the effects of this food on your body.

The rest of this book contains a collection of recipes to give you an idea of the kinds of things you can enjoy for breakfast, lunch, dinner and snacks.

RECIPES
Breakfast

Breakfast Burgers

1 lb ground pork
1 tsp sea salt
1 tsp dried sage
1 tsp dried thyme
1/2 tsp ground ginger
1/2 tsp dried rosemary

1) Place the pork in a large bowl and add the salt, sage, thyme, ginger and rosemary. Mix well.

2) Separate out the mixture into 4 x 4 oz portions and mold each portion into the shape of a burger patty.

3) Put each patty on a flat board and freeze until just firm to the touch. Remove the frozen patties from the board and store the ones that you don't want to cook yet.

4) Cook the patties in a frying pan over a medium heat and until brown on both sides and fully cooked.

Fruit Boost Smoothie

1 medium banana, chopped
1 apple, cored and quartered
1 inch root ginger, peeled
2 peaches, chopped
1/4 lemon, peeled
1/2 cup water
1 tbsp olive oil

1) Blend all ingredients in an electric mixer or blender, and serve immediately.

Lunch

Pumpkin Soup

1 medium butternut squash, peeled and chopped
1 medium onion, peeled and chopped
2 stalks celery, chopped
2 cloves garlic, crushed
6 cups organic chicken or vegetable stock
1 large orange, juiced
Pinch of salt and black pepper

1) Heat the oil in a large saucepan and cook the pumpkin, onion, celery and garlic for 5 minutes at a medium heat.

2) Add the stock to the saucepan and cover. Cook for a further 25-30 minutes.

3) Blend the contents of the saucepan until of a smooth consistency.

4) Return to the saucepan and season with salt, pepper and orange juice.

5) Can be served hot or cold.

Chicken and Avocado Ranch Salad

2 cups romaine lettuce, chopped
1/2 cup carrots, shredded

1/2 cup red bell pepper, sliced
3 oz chicken breast, grilled and sliced
1/4 avocado, mashed
1 1/2 tbsp organic ranch dressing

1) Add the romaine lettuce, carrots, bell pepper and chicken to a bowl.

2) Mash the avocado with the ranch dressing.

3) Add the dressing to the salad, toss and serve.

Dinner

Indian-inspired Chicken and Lentil Soup

1 tsp olive oil

1/2 medium onion, chopped

1 inch piece of root ginger

3 garlic cloves, chopped

2 green chillies (optional)

1/2 tsp ground turmeric

1 tsp salt

1/2 tsp ground cumin

150 grams split green lentils

1 liter organic chicken stock

3 1/2 oz chicken breast, skinned, poached and diced

1 tbsp lemon juice

2 tbsp fresh cilantro

1) Heat the olive oil in a saucepan.

2) Sauté the onion for 1 minute at a medium heat.

3) Add the ginger, garlic and chillies, and sauté.

4) Add the turmeric, salt, ground cumin, lentils and chicken stock to the saucepan. Cook at medium heat for 15 minutes. Pass through a sieve and return to the saucepan.

5) Add the diced chicken to the mixture, and bring it to the boil. Add water if necessary.

6) Continue to simmer for 2-3 minutes and add the lemon juice.

7) Serve hot with a garnish of cilantro leaves.

Cauliflower Ratatouille

5 1/2 oz cauliflower florets

9 oz mixed bell peppers, deseeded and chopped

2 oz red onion, thinly sliced

2 oz zucchini, chopped

1 tbsp thyme leaves

1 tbsp rosemary leaves

Olive oil

Pinch of salt and black pepper

Chopped parsley

1) Preheat the oven to 400 degrees F.

2) Blanch the cauliflower in a saucepan of boiling water. Drain, rinse in cold water and pat dry.

3) Place the vegetables on a baking tray and drizzle with olive oil.

4) Add the chopped thyme and rosemary, and season with salt and pepper.

5) Roast the vegetables for 15-20 minutes until golden brown. Turn them halfway through.

6) Serve with freshly chopped parsley to garnish.

Snacks

Vegetable Guacamole

2 avocados
1/2 cucumber, diced
1/2 yellow squash, grated
1/2 zucchini, grated
1 clove of garlic, minced
Juice from half a lime
Fresh cilantro, chopped
Sea salt
Wedge of lime

1) Mash the avocados and mix all the ingredients in a bowl.

2) Garnish with a lime wedge.

Pickled Gherkins

25 small cucumbers
1/2 lb salt
2 quarts water
0.6 quarts white vinegar
1 tbsp pickling spice

1) Add the salt to the water to make brine.

2) Cover the cucumbers with the brine in a large pan.

3) Heat the liquid to near boiling point, but do not actually boil. Simmer for 10 minutes.

4) Drain the cucumbers and allow to cool.

5) Place the vinegar and pickling spice in a saucepan and bring to the boil for 1 minute.

6) Pack the cucumbers into a warm Kilner jar, and cover with the vinegar.

7) These pickles can be stored for weeks and eaten as a snack whenever you like.

Pineapple and Basil Smoothie

1/2 cup pineapple, chopped
1/8 inch root ginger, peeled
1/2 medium banana, chopped
1/2 cup coconut milk
1 tbsp fresh basil, chopped

1) Blend ingredients in an electric mixer or blender, and serve immediately.

Conclusion

Thank you for reading this full book. I have written all the information about 'Myasthenia Gravis'. Don't be frustrated about Myasthenia Gravis. Knowledge can go a long way in treatment and prevention.

Made in the USA
Middletown, DE
24 April 2025

74721500R00027